Y1 363

ST. MARY'S & ST. PETER'S
C/E PRIMARY SCHOOL
SOMERSET ROAD
TEDDINGTON
081-943 0476

3812

D1588697

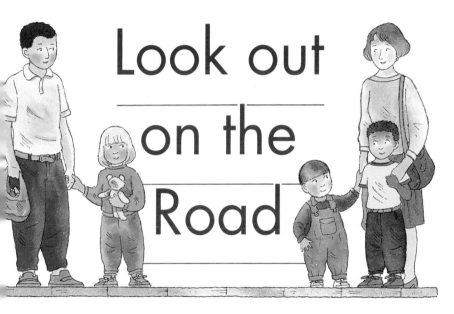

Look out
on the
Road

Paul Humphrey and
Alex Ramsay

Illustrated by
Colin King

Evans

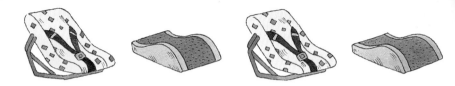

We're going shopping and then we can go for a walk in the country.

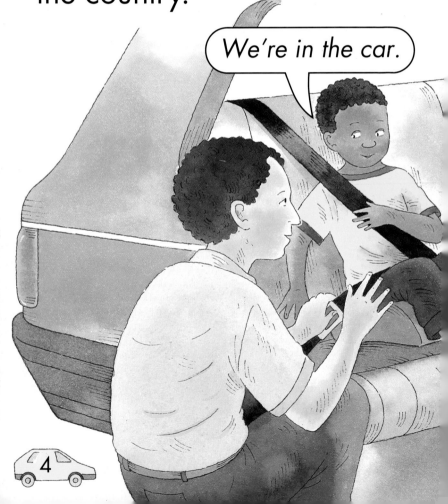

We're in the car.

4

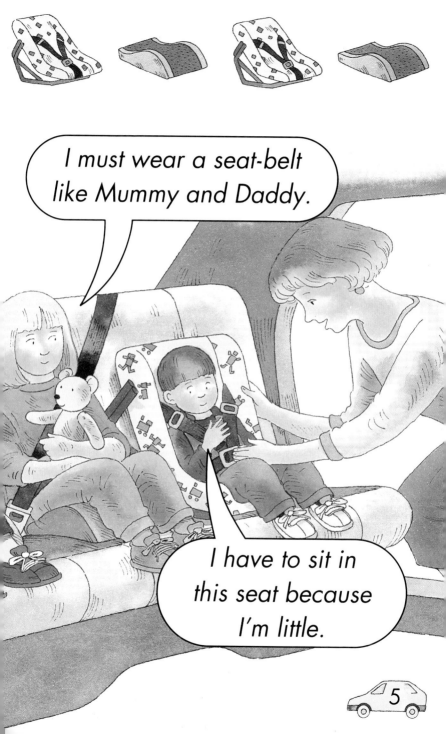

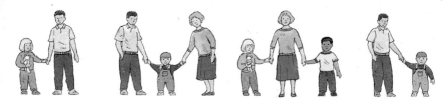

Here we are at the shops.

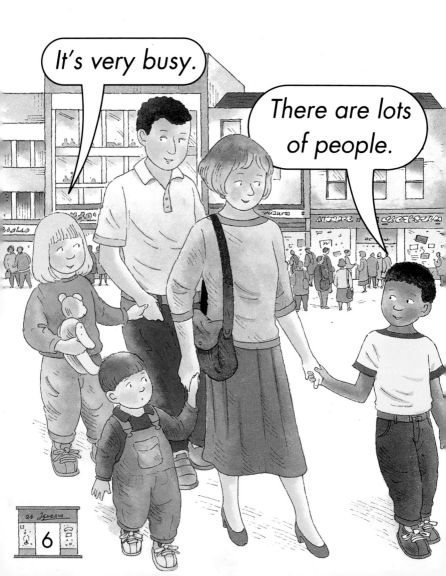

6

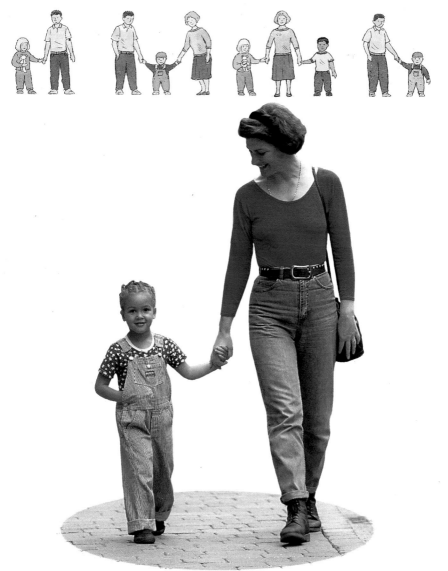

Always hold a grown-up's
hand, then you will be safe.

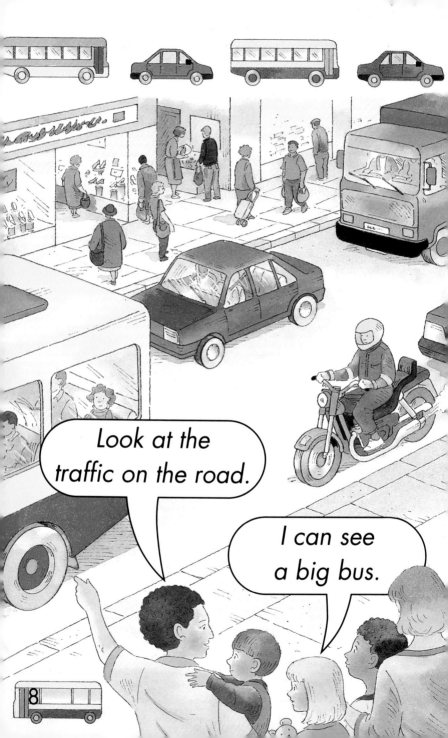

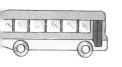 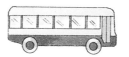

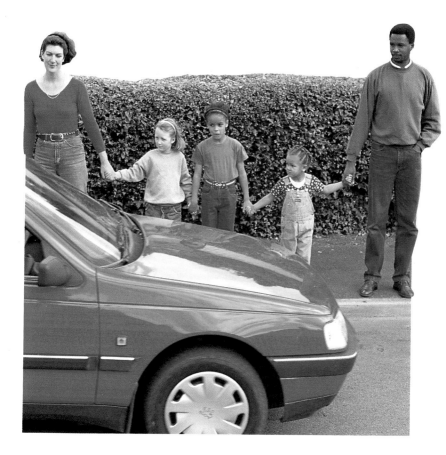

Always be careful when
you are near a road.

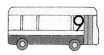

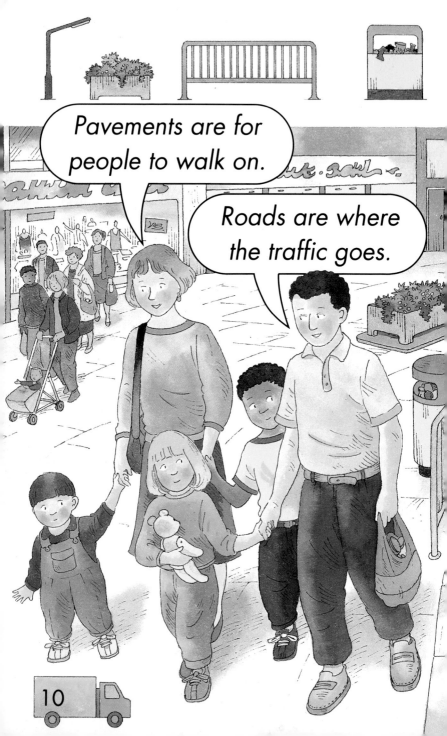

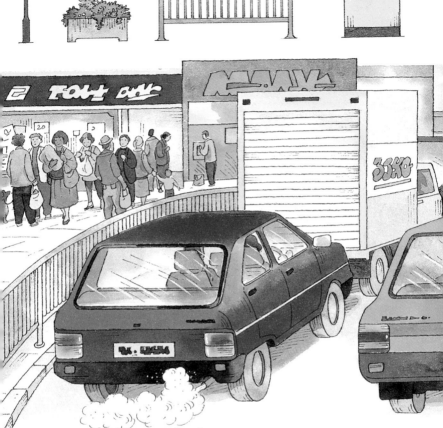

The edge of the pavement
is called the kerb.
Never stand too close
to the kerb.

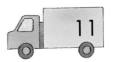

11

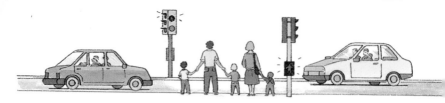

Let's look for a safe place to cross the road.
Here is a pelican crossing.

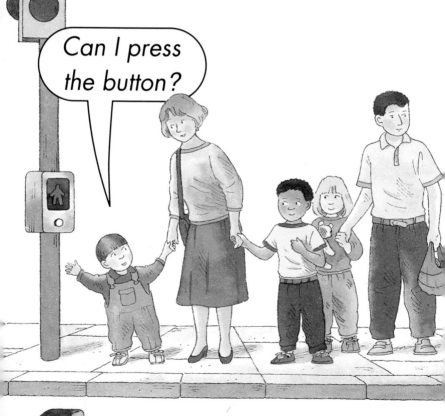

Can I press the button?

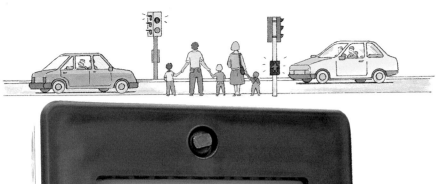

PEDESTRIANS
push button and wait for signal opposite

WAIT

wait | cross with care | do not start to cross

FLASHING

13

Now we must wait for the signal before we cross the road.

I can see the red man.

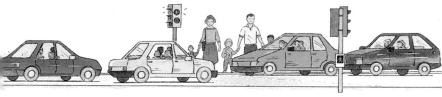

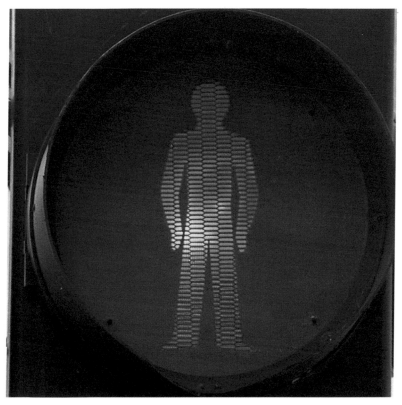

The red man shows us
that it's not safe to cross
the road.

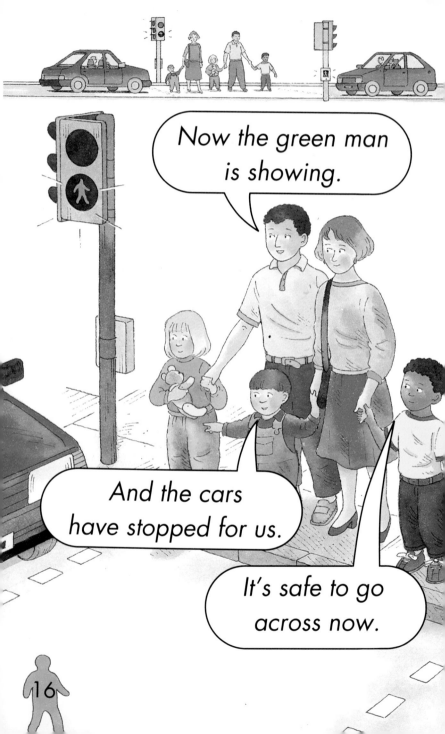

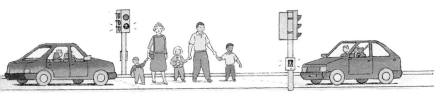

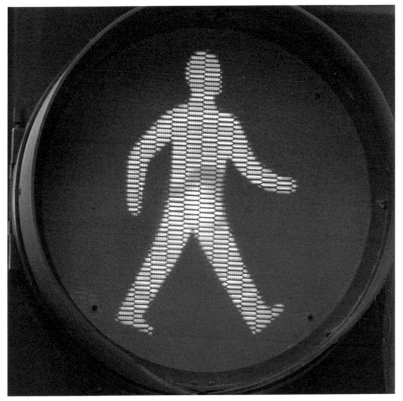

Be sure to go on looking and
listening while you cross
the road.

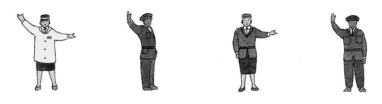

There are other safe places
to cross the road.

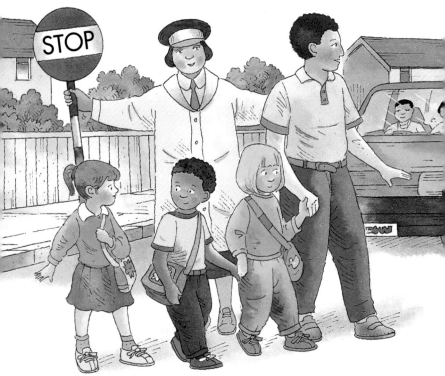

The lollipop lady at school
stops the traffic.

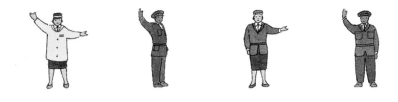

Policemen sometimes help
people to cross the road.

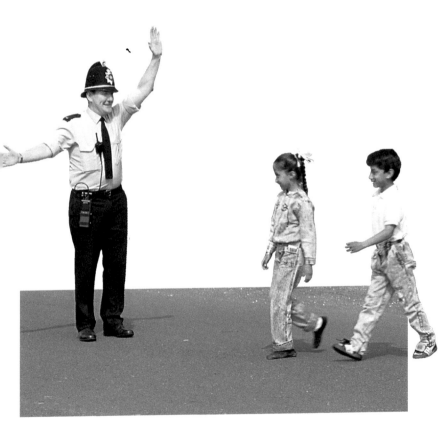

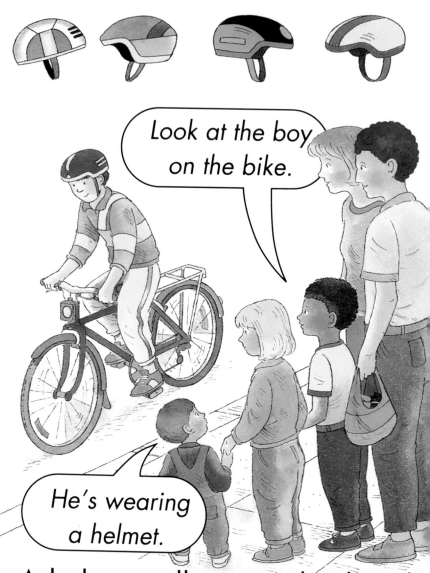

A helmet will protect his head
if he falls off his bike.

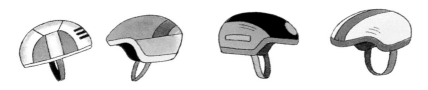

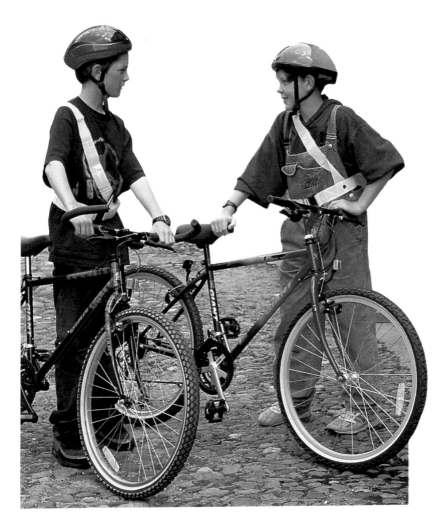

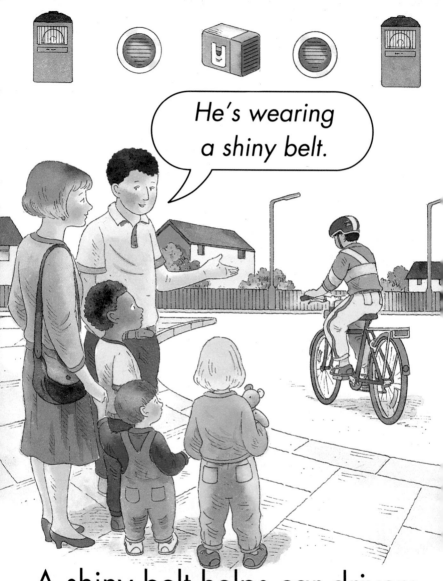

A shiny belt helps car drivers
to see him easily.

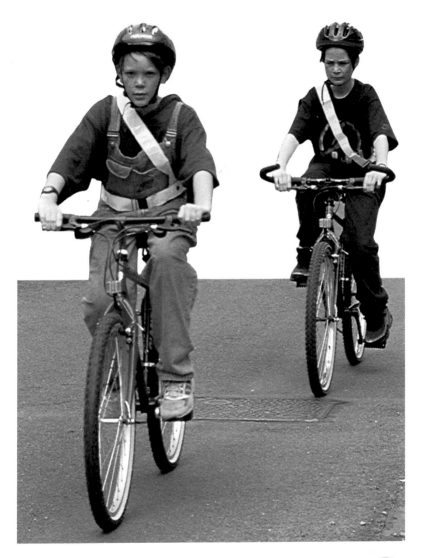

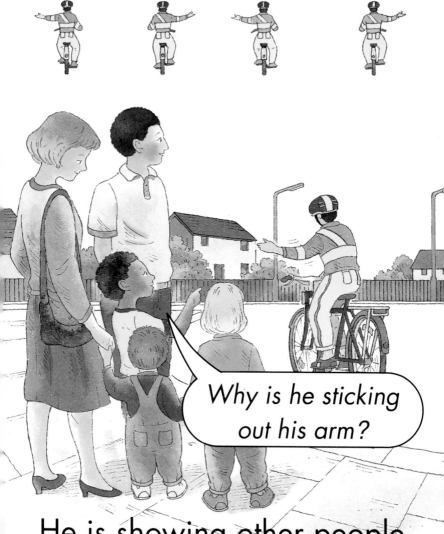

Why is he sticking out his arm?

He is showing other people on the road that he wants to turn left.

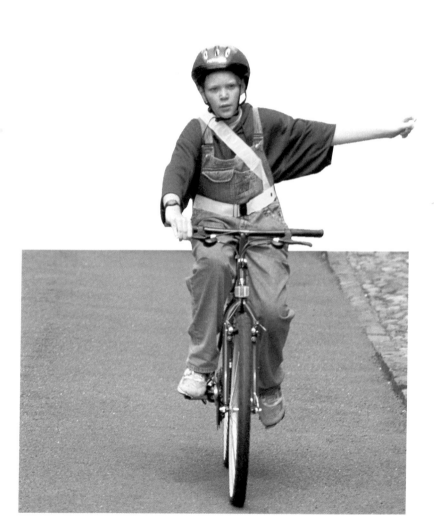

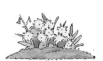

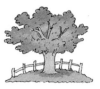

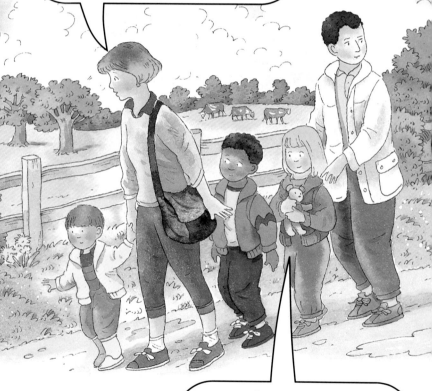

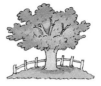

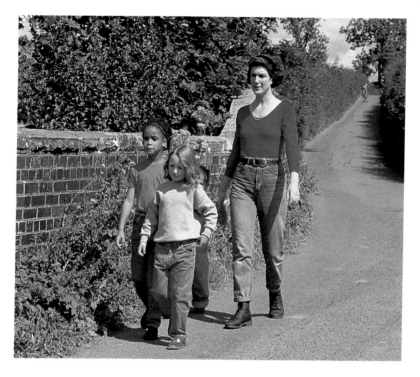

Always walk on the
right-hand side of the
road so that you can be
seen by the traffic.

Can you remember
the rules for crossing
the road
safely?

Always STOP
at the kerb.

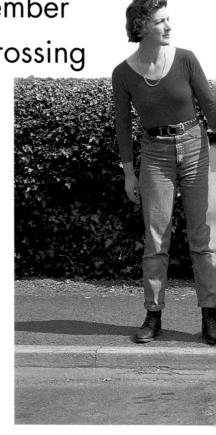

LOOK out for traffic.

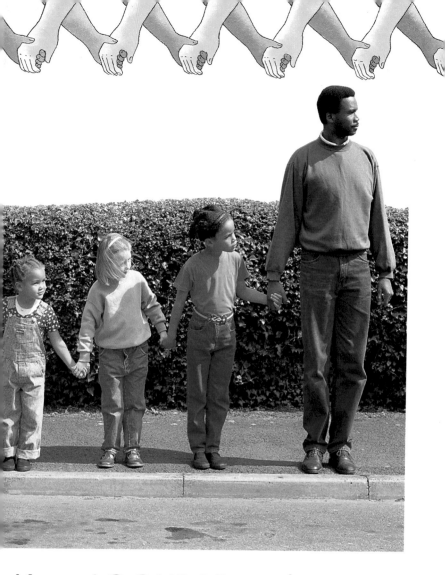

Keep LOOKING and
LISTENING as you cross.

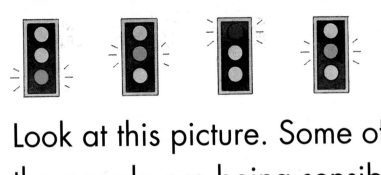

Look at this picture. Some of the people are being sensible and some are being silly. Which are which?